PERFECTING GUT HEALTH

Gut Health Products You Should Know

James Edwards

TABLE OF CONTENTS

INTRODUCTION

The critical role that gut health plays in overall health and vigor has come to light more and more in recent years. Our total health is greatly impacted by the state of our digestive system, from daily strength to the avoidance of chronic illnesses. The goal of this book is to provide you with a thorough grasp of gut health, its significance, and the items available to support your gut health.

Plenty of microorganisms, such as bacteria, viruses, and fungi, live in the human gut, which is an ever-changing and intricate nature. The immune system, digestion, nutritional absorption, and mental health are all significantly impacted by this microbiome. On the other hand, the precise harmony of these microorganisms in the gut can be upset by modern lives, which are marked by poor food, stress, and abuse of antibiotics, resulting in a variety of health problems. Becoming aware of how your gut functions and what it requires to be healthy is the starting point of enjoying improved health.

A healthy gut not only serves for efficient digestion but also as a guard, keeping dangerous things out of the body and enabling the body to absorb essential nutrients. Furthermore, the gut-brain axis illustrates how mood, stress levels, and mental ability are all significantly impacted by the state of gut health. Numerous illnesses, such as diabetes, heart disease, obesity, and autoimmune disorders are associated with gut health, according to recent studies. Thus, the cornerstone of general health and energy is preserving the health of the gut.

With so many alternatives accessible today, it can be difficult to make a quality decision in relation to gut health products. By offering thorough explanations of a wide range of products, including fermented foods, digestive enzymes, probiotics, and prebiotics, this book seeks to clarify this complex field. We will go over the advantages, possible side effects, and the best ways to use these products in your regular routine. We'll also dig into the science underlying these products so you can make quality decisions based on the most recent studies.

This book serves as your manual for comprehending and perfecting your gut health. It doesn't matter if you're just a health enthusiast seeking to expand your knowledge or a person experiencing digestive problems, this book provides insightful analysis and useful guidance to help you live a happier, longer life. Let us progress to uncover the mysteries of a gut that is in perfect harmony, which is one of the primary keys to ultimate health.

CHAPTER ONE

The Fundamentals of Probiotics as A Gut Health Product

Gastrointestinal health frequently becomes the focus of attention in the pursuit of ideal health. A healthy gut affects everything from the immune system to digestion to mental health, and it is essential for general comfort. Probiotics are one of the most effective and well-known preferences for improving gut health among the plethora of options accessible. In this chapter, we shall be focusing on understanding the things that probiotics are all about, their health benefits, and common sources of probiotics.

Definition of Probiotics

Probiotics are functioning bacteria that give humans health benefits when taken in sufficient quantities. For this reason, they are frequently referred to as "friendly" or "good" bacteria since they support gut health. Although your body naturally contains these advantageous bacteria, you can also consume some of the food and supplements that contain them.

The majority of probiotics are found in the gut, especially in the large intestine, where they are essential for preserving the equilibrium of the gut flora. Appropriate digestion, absorption of nutrients, and immune system response depend on this equilibrium.

Six Major Health Benefits of Probiotics

Probiotics provide advantages that go beyond digestive health. Here are the six major health benefits:

1. Better Digestive Health: A balanced population of gut bacteria is necessary for effective digestion, and probiotics can support this equilibrium. They can reduce the symptoms of gastrointestinal conditions like diarrhea, irritable bowel syndrome (IBS), and inflammatory bowel disease (IBD), which could arise as a result of infections or antibiotics.

2. Stronger Immune Function: The gut contains a substantial part of the immune system. By encouraging the creation of natural antibodies and preventing the growth of pathogenic bacteria, probiotics can improve the immune response.

3. Improved Nutrient Absorption: Probiotics help to promote the absorption of vital nutrients, such as vitamins and minerals, by preserving a healthy gut environment.

4. Better Mental Health Condition: The gut-brain axis is a sophisticated network of communication that connects the two organs. This relationship has been demonstrated to be influenced by probiotics, which may lessen the signs of anxiety, depression, and other mental health issues.

5. Weight Control: Research indicates that probiotics may impact how the body stores fat, as well as controlling hunger and energy levels, to aid with weight control.

6. Lessened Eczema and Allergies: Probiotics, especially in youngsters, may help lessen the incidence and intensity of eczema and allergies.

Seven Major Sources of Probiotics

Probiotics are becoming more and more popular, and as a result, the market is overflowing with options. Here are seven highly recommended probiotic sources to take into account:

1. Yogurt: Packed with living and active cultures that help promote gut health, yogurt is one of the most popular forms of probiotics. For maximum benefits, look for goods labeled with 'live and active cultures'.

2. Kefir: Rich in calcium and protein, this fermented milk beverage is loaded with probiotics. Kefir is a fantastic dietary meal for improving gastrointestinal well-being.

3. Sauerkraut: A great source of fiber, vitamins, and probiotics, sauerkraut is fermented cabbage. It's a delightful and nourishing method of improving your gut health.

4. Kimchi: A common Korean meal prepared from fermented vegetables, kimchi is rich in minerals and vitamins A, B, and C in addition to being a potent source of probiotics.

5. Kombucha: This is a fermented tea that is popular as a good source of probiotics, helping to support better digestion and a stronger immune system.

6. Miso: This is a Japanese seasoning that is rich in probiotics. It is derived from fermented soybeans, and it imparts a distinct flavor to soups, marinades, and sauces.

7. Probiotic Supplements: Supplements are an easy alternative solution for people who might not get sufficient probiotics from meals alone. It's important to seek premium products with a high colony-forming unit (CFU) count and a range of probiotic strains.

In summary, probiotics have many advantages that exceed their usefulness in the digestive system, making them an essential part of gut health. Adding foods or supplements that are high in probiotics to your daily diet can assist in keeping your gastrointestinal flora in a healthy state, strengthening your immune system, and improving your general health. It's important for you to understand that all probiotics are not made equal, so endeavor to make informed decisions as you consider the best source of probiotics to embrace, as you strive to perfect your gut health.

CHAPTER TWO

The Fundamentals of Prebiotics as A Gut Health Product

Prebiotics are indigestible food ingredients that improve the health of the gut by selectively promoting either the growth or activity of a single or small group of bacteria within the colon of the intestinal tract. Prebiotics are basically food substances that nourish probiotics, which are functioning beneficial bacteria in the gut. Their principal constituents include resistant starches and a variety of fibers that are indigestible to human digestive enzymes but travel to the colon via the digestive tract, where the gut flora ferments them.

Five Principal Advantages of Prebiotics

1. Better Digestive Health: Prebiotics encourage the development of useful bacteria, like lactobacilli and bifidobacteria, which can support the maintenance of a balanced gut flora. Maintaining this equilibrium is essential for efficient digestion and averting gastrointestinal ailments such as inflammatory bowel disease (IBD) and irritable bowel syndrome (IBS).

2. Stronger Immunity: The gut contains a substantial part of the immune system. Prebiotics support a healthy gut flora, which strengthens the immune system and increases its capacity to fight off infections and illnesses.

3. Improved Nutrient Absorption: Prebiotics can improve the body's ability to absorb vital nutrients like calcium and magnesium from the diet by fostering the

growth of useful bacteria. These mineral substances assist in maintaining stronger bones and improving the body's general health.

4. Decreased Inflammation: The body's overall inflammation can be decreased with the support of a healthy gut flora. This effect of decreased inflammation is very useful because numerous medical conditions, such as diabetes, heart disease, and several types of cancer, are associated with chronic inflammation.

5. Better Metabolic Health: Research has indicated that prebiotics affect the synthesis of hormones that control appetite and fat storage. This may result in better weight control and a lower chance of obesity-related illnesses.

Ten Major Sources of Prebiotics

Maintaining a healthy gut flora can be achieved by including a range of foods that are high in prebiotics in your diet. The top ten sources are as follows:

1. Chicory Root: This is one of the best sources of inulin, which is a kind of prebiotic fiber that promotes digestive health. Chicory root is frequently used as an alternative to coffee.

2. Garlic: In addition to its spicy use, garlic is rich in fructooligosaccharides (FOS) and inulin, which encourage the growth of health-promoting Bifidobacteria in the gastrointestinal tract.

3. Onions: Another great source of fructooligosaccharides (FOS) and inulin is onions. Additionally, they contain quercetin, an anti-inflammatory antioxidant.

4. Leeks: Packed with inulin and fructooligosaccharides (FOS), leeks are an excellent way to add extra prebiotic nutrition to soups, stews, and salads. They are similar to onions and garlic in this regard.

5. Asparagus: Asparagus offers vital vitamins and minerals and has a high inulin content, which supports gut health.

6. Bananas: Resistant starch, especially from green bananas, functions as a prebiotic by nourishing useful bacteria in the gut to support gut health.

7. Jerusalem Artichokes: Also referred to as sunchokes, these inulin-rich tubers can be added to a range of meals to increase the amount of fiber that is consumed.

8. Dandelion Greens: It is frequently employed in making salads, and it's rich in inulin and fiber, which promote healthy liver and digestive systems.

9. Barley: It is a whole grain that contains a form of fiber called beta-glucan, which functions as a prebiotic. It can be employed in making salads, stews, and soups.

10. Oats: It consists of both beta-glucan and resistant starch, which have prebiotic properties. They can be employed in making oatmeal, baked products, or as a component of a well-balanced diet.

Four Vital Tips for Including Prebiotics in Your Daily Diet

Eating a range of meals high in prebiotics on a daily basis is crucial to maximizing the importance of prebiotics. The following four tips are essential for adding prebiotics to your diet:

a. Bring Variety to Your Diet: To guarantee a well-rounded intake of diverse fibers and resistant starches, try to incorporate a variety of prebiotic sources into your diet.

b. Combine Probiotics and Prebiotics: You can increase the potency of probiotic-rich foods like yogurt, kefir, and fermented vegetables by consuming prebiotic foods along with them.

c. Begin Gradually: In order to avoid stomach pain, if you're not used to eating high-fiber foods, start consuming them at a steady pace.

d. Remain Hydrated: Fiber passes more easily in the digestive system when you drink a lot of water.

In summary, prebiotics are essential for preserving a balanced gut flora, which promotes general health and comfort. You may support long-term health and nourish your gut by learning about the advantages of prebiotics and including a range of foods high in prebiotics in your diet.

CHAPTER THREE

The Fundamentals of Fermented Foods as A Gut Health Product

For generations, fermented foods have been a nourishment in many cultures, valued for their distinct tastes and health advantages. Microorganisms such as bacteria, yeast, and molds naturally transform sugars and starch into acids or alcohol through a process called fermentation. This procedure improves the food's digestion and nutritional composition in addition to aiding in preservation. Fermented foods are important because they introduce useful probiotics, which are functioning bacteria that promote healthy gut flora.

Our digestive system is home to a complex colony of numerous microorganisms called the gut flora. For the best possible digestion, nutritional absorption, immune system performance, as well as mental wellness, a healthy gut flora is necessary. Fermented foods promote a healthy gut flora in the following ways:

1. Increasing Intake of Probiotics: They are abundant in probiotics, which can aid in supplying and balancing the gut flora.

2. Improving the Absorption of Nutrients: Fermentation can raise a nutrient's bioavailability, which facilitates our bodies' ability to absorb it.

3. Boosting Immune Function: Fermented foods can support the balance of a healthy gut flora, which is associated with a more robust immune system.

4. Improving Digestion: Fermented foods promote digestion, decreasing bloating and gas, since the enzymes created during fermentation assist the body to break down complex carbohydrates and proteins that otherwise would have led to bloating and gas.

Seven Major Sources of Fermented Food

1. Yogurt: This is probably the top famous fermented food. It is formed by adding bacterial cultures to milk to ferment it. It contains a lot of probiotics, including strains of Lactobacillus and Bifidobacterium. In addition, yogurt has significant levels of protein, calcium, and vitamins B12 and B2.

2. Kefir: This is a fermented milk beverage that resembles yogurt but has a wider variety of probiotics and a thinner consistency. It is a powerful source of probiotics because it has up to 30 different types of bacteria and helpful yeasts. In addition, Kefir has significant levels of vitamins and minerals such as calcium, magnesium, and phosphorus.

3. Sauerkraut: This is a common nourishment in many European meals. It is produced from fermented cabbage. It contains a lot of useful bacteria, such as Leuconostoc mesenteroides and Lactobacillus plantarum. In addition, Kefir has significant levels of fiber, vitamin C, and vitamin K.

4. Kimchi: This is a fermented vegetable food that is common in Korea. It is produced from radishes and napa cabbage mixed with a variety of flavors. It is renowned for having a sharp and peppery flavor. Apart from containing abundant probiotics, Kimchi also contains vitamins A, B, C, and important minerals.

5. Miso: This is a common condiment in Japan. It is made by using a fungus called Aspergillus oryzae and salt to ferment soybeans. It's generally used in marinades,

sauces, and soups. Miso contains useful bacteria such as Bifidobacterium and Lactobacillus, and it's rich in protein, vitamins, and minerals.

6. Tempeh: This is a fermented soybean product that originated from Indonesia. It tastes like nuts and has a hard texture. Tempeh is a great source of probiotics, as well as fiber and protein. It is a fantastic meat substitute for vegetarians and vegans because, apart from the protein and fiber it constitutes, it also contains enough vitamins B2, B6, and B12.

7. Kombucha: This is a fermented tea drink that is produced by fermenting sweetened tea with a symbiotic culture of bacteria and yeast (SCOBY). Kombucha is somewhat foamy, and it can be spiced up with fruits and herbs. It contains lots of probiotics, as well as antioxidants and vitamins, especially the B vitamins.

Six Practical Tips for Including Fermented Foods in Your Daily Diet

It can be pleasurable and useful for the health of your gut to include fermented foods in your diet. Here are six practical tips that can assist you:

1. Begin Gradually: In order to avoid stomach pain, if you're not used to eating fermented foods, start consuming them at a steady pace. As your body adjusts, you can keep increasing the portions gradually.

2. Expand Your Options: To get the benefits of various probiotic strains and diverse nutrients, introduce various fermented foods to your diet. Try some kimchi or sauerkraut for lunch, yogurt for breakfast, and a cup of kombucha for dessert.

3. Integrate with Meals: You can easily include fermented foods in your meals. Use miso in soups, yogurt or kefir in smoothies, or tempeh as a source of protein in salads and stir-fries.

4. Flirt with Cooking Directions: Use your imagination to prepare new dishes that include fermented foods. Try your hand at making your own kefir and yogurt, or prepare kimchi or sauerkraut for yourself.

5. Read Labels: Look for goods that include live, active cultures when buying fermented foods. Steer clear of those that have artificial substances or additional sweets since these can counteract any health and wellness benefits.

6. Continuous Effort Yields Results: Continuous consumption of fermented foods is essential for perfecting gut health. Make it a point to eat a minimum of one portion of fermented food every day.

In summary, eating fermented foods is a tasty and practical approach to perfect gut health. Including a range of these foods high in probiotics in your diet can improve immune system function, aid with digestion, and generally improve your health. On your path to optimal gut health, adopt the habit of consuming tasty and sustaining fermented foods.

CHAPTER FOUR

The Fundamentals of Fiber-Rich Foods as A Gut Health Product

Consuming dietary fiber is essential to preserving the best possible gut health. Fiber, which is sometimes disregarded, is essential for maintaining healthy digestive tract operations as well as general well-being. This chapter explores the benefits of eating foods high in fiber for gut health, the major sources of dietary fiber, and the significance of fiber supplements.

The indigestible portion of plant meals that passes through our digestive systems, absorbing water along the way and facilitating bowel movements is called dietary fiber. They are sometimes referred to as roughage. Dietary fiber comes in two varieties with different benefits, and they include soluble and insoluble fibers.

1. Soluble Fiber: This type of dietary fiber turns into a gel-like material when it dissolves in water. It assists in the reduction of both cholesterol and blood sugar. Common sources of soluble fiber include carrots, barley, beans, peas, citrus fruits, psyllium, and apples.

2. Insoluble Fiber: This type of fiber makes stools bulkier and facilitates the passage of materials through the digestive tract. It helps people who experience irregular or constipated feces. Common sources of insoluble fiber include wheat bran, whole-wheat flour, legumes, nuts, and vegetables like potatoes, cauliflower, and green beans.

Five Major Benefits of Dietary Fiber to Gut Health:

1. Discourages Constipation: Fiber softens and makes your stool heavier and bigger. The likelihood of constipation is reduced when the stool is thick and easy to pass.

2. Promotes Bowel Health: Eating a diet rich in fiber may reduce your danger of acquiring hemorrhoids and small pouches (diverticular disease) in your colon. A diet that is rich in fiber is also thought to reduce the incidence of colorectal cancer, according to research.

3. Lowers Cholesterol Levels: By lowering bad cholesterol (LDL) levels, soluble fiber, which is present in beans, oats, flaxseed, and oat bran, may help lower overall blood cholesterol levels.

4. Aids in Managing Blood Sugar Levels: Fiber, especially soluble fiber, can lower blood sugar levels by slowing the absorption of sugar. Insoluble fiber from a balanced diet may help lower the chance of type 2 diabetes.

5. Promotes Healthy Weight Goal: Because high-fiber foods are higher in calories and more satisfying than low-fiber foods, you'll probably eat less and feel fuller for longer. Foods high in fiber typically have a lower "energy density," or fewer calories per serving, and require longer time to consume.

Five Major Sources of Dietary Fiber

Perfecting gut health requires including a range of foods high in fiber in your diet. The following are the top five dietary fiber sources:

1. Fruits: Both soluble and insoluble fibers are present in some fruits, such as bananas, and they aid in digestion. Strawberries, blackberries, and raspberries are a few examples of berries that are high in fiber. Pears and apples, especially with the skin retained, are a good source of dietary fiber.

2. Vegetables: Examples of vegetables include carrots, broccoli, and Brussels sprouts. Carrots are rich sources of fiber and antioxidants. Broccoli is well-known for its high fiber content and advantages for intestinal health. Brussels sprouts contain lots of vitamins, minerals, and fiber.

3. Legumes: Black beans, chickpeas, and lentils are a few types of legumes. Black beans are rich in nutrients and fiber. Chickpeas are an excellent addition to salads and soups due to their versatility and high fiber content. Lentils are incredibly high in protein and fiber.

4. Whole Grains: Oats, brown rice, and quinoa are a few types of whole grains. There's a large quantity of insoluble fiber in brown rice. Oats and Quinoa contain soluble fiber and protein and fiber respectively.

5. Nuts and Seeds: Almonds, flaxseeds, and chia seeds are a few types of nuts and seeds. Almonds are a fantastic, high-fiber snack choice. An excellent balance of soluble and insoluble fiber can be found in flaxseeds. Chia seeds have a very high fiber content, both insoluble and soluble varieties.

Four Common Types of Fiber Supplements

Although consuming fiber through food is ideal, if you are having problems getting adequate fiber from your diet, fiber supplements may be helpful. Four popular kinds of fiber supplements are as follows:

1. Psyllium Husk: This is a soluble fiber that is sourced from Plantago ovata seeds and is frequently used to relieve constipation and promote digestive health.

2. Methylcellulose: This is a water-soluble synthetic fiber that is derived from cellulose. It can be used to relieve constipation, as well as alleviate irregular bowel movements.

3. Inulin: This is a soluble fiber that is present in plants and serves as a prebiotic by nourishing the beneficial bacteria or probiotics in your digestive system.

4. Wheat Dextrin: This is a soluble fiber that is sourced from wheat starch. It is normally found in supplements such as Benefiber.

Three Major Benefits of Fiber Supplements

1. Convenience: Simple to include in everyday activities, particularly for people with hectic schedules.

2. Customizable Dosage: Fiber intake can be regulated and customized to meet specific demands by virtue of supplements.

3. Aid for Certain Conditions: Helpful in reducing the symptoms of illnesses like high cholesterol, constipation, and IBS.

Three Crucial Cautions when Taking Supplemental Fiber

1. Hydration: To avoid constipation when taking fiber supplements, drink more water.

2. Gradual Introduction: To prevent gastrointestinal distress, introduce fiber supplements gradually.

3. Seek Professional Counsel: Before beginning any new supplement regimen, especially if you have hidden medical concerns, always get advice from a healthcare professional.

Finally, adding fiber to your diet is an easy yet really powerful strategy to perfect your gut health. There are many options to fit all tastes and nutritional preferences among the range of fiber-rich foods available, ranging from whole fruits and vegetables to legumes and whole grains. Supplements with fiber can also be helpful if needed. You will be making a very big step toward perfecting your gut health when you make dietary fiber a priority.

CHAPTER FIVE

The Fundamental Knowledge of Digestive Enzymes Towards Perfecting Gut Health

Digestive enzymes are proteins that help the digestive tract absorb nutrients by catalyzing the breakdown of food to absorbable nutrients. They guarantee that the body gets the nutrients it needs from meals to function at its best and are crucial for healthy digestion and nutrient absorption. There are different kinds of digestive enzymes, each focusing on a certain macronutrient:

1. Proteases: It functions to disintegrate proteins into their constituent amino acids.

2. Lipases: It functions to convert lipids or fats into glycerol and fatty acids.

3. Amylases: It functions to convert carbohydrates into monosaccharides.

4. Lactase: It functions to disintegrate lactose, the milk sugar, to its simplest absorbable unit.

5. Cellulase: It functions to disintegrate cellulose, the fiber in plants, to its simplest absorbable unit.

The pancreas, stomach, and small intestine are the main organs that manufacture these enzymes, and they are all essential to the digestion process.

Five Major Benefits of Digestive Enzymes for Gut Health

There are several uses of digestive enzymes for gut health and general comfort, and they include:

1. Better Digestion: By aiding in the more effective disintegration of food, enzymes lower the risk of gas, bloating, and indigestion.

2. Improved Nutrient Absorption: Digestive enzymes help the body absorb more nutrients by disintegrating food into smaller, more absorbable units, which guarantees the body gets the vital vitamins, minerals, and other elements it needs.

3. Reduction of Food Intolerance Symptoms: By giving people with certain food intolerances — like lactose intolerance — the enzymes they need to disintegrate these foods, enzyme supplements can assist in reducing food intolerance symptoms.

4. Promotion of Pancreatic Health: Taking digestive enzyme supplements can lessen the task on the pancreas, which is especially advantageous for those who suffer from pancreatic insufficiency or other pancreatic diseases.

5. Reduction of Digestive Disorders: Enzyme supplements may help people with digestive disorders such as irritable bowel syndrome (IBS), Celiac disease, and Crohn's disease by reducing their symptoms.

The Top Five Supplements for Digestive Enzymes

The health of the digestive system can be greatly impacted by the choice of a premium digestive enzyme supplement. These are the top five enzyme supplements on the market right now:

1. Zenwise Health Digestive Enzymes with Prebiotics & Probiotics: Peptide, amylase, lipase, and cellulase are among the many enzymes included in this all-inclusive blend. It is also supplemented with probiotics and prebiotics for further benefits to gut health. As such, it fits a variety of dietary requirements and eases discomfort and bloating.

2. Enzymedica Digest Gold with ATPro: This is one of the strongest enzyme formulae on the market. It is made up of a broad variety of enzymes that focus on fibers, proteins, lipids, and carbohydrates. The ATPro blend promotes the generation of energy and facilitates the effective use of nutrients.

3. NOW Super Enzymes: This supplement provides complete digestive support by combining a potent blend of enzymes with pancreatin, ox bile, and betaine HCl. It is especially helpful for people who have gallbladder problems or low stomach acid. It aids in the breakdown of carbohydrates, lipids, and proteins.

4. Garden of Life Vegetarian Digestive Supplement: This enzyme supplement made of plants is perfect for vegans and vegetarians. It includes specific enzymes for the digestion of dairy and gluten, as well as general enzymes like lipase, amylase, and protease. It is supplemented with minerals and trace elements to promote general digestive system support.

5. Pure Encapsulations Digestive Enzymes Ultra: This hypoallergenic formula is appropriate for people with delicate digestive systems. It offers a complete blend of enzymes for total support of the digestive system. Because of its excellent quality and purity, medical practitioners recognize it as a reliable option.

In summary, the presence of digestive enzymes is essential for preserving gut health and guaranteeing effective digestion and absorption of nutrients. Digestive enzyme supplements can be quite useful, particularly for people with certain dietary intolerances or digestive issues. When selecting a digestive enzyme supplement, it's critical to take into account the particular enzymes present, the product's quality, and any extra substances that can increase its efficacy. You may promote your digestive health and general comfort by adding the appropriate digestive enzyme supplement to your regimen, which will help in your pursuit of perfect gut health.

CHAPTER SIX

The Fundamental Knowledge of Herbal Supplements for Gut Health

Boosting gut health with herbs has become more and more popular as a natural and efficient way to perfect gut health. This chapter explores the realm of herbal therapies for gut health, looking at both the efficacy and safety of common herbal supplements.

Five Major Herbs for Gut Health

For generations, traditional medicine has employed herbs to promote digestive health. Their inherent qualities can lessen inflammation, calm the digestive system, and enhance general gut health. Here are five popular herbs that are well-known for improving gut health:

1. Peppermint: Peppermint has a well-established reputation for relieving gastrointestinal distress. Its primary component, menthol, possesses antispasmodic qualities that aid in calming the gastrointestinal tract's muscles and lessening irritable bowel syndrome (IBS) symptoms like gas, bloating, and abdominal pain.

2. Ginger: For centuries, ginger has been utilized to relieve indigestion and nausea. It possesses anti-inflammatory and antioxidant qualities that can aid in lowering gut inflammation, enhancing digestion, and easing gastrointestinal discomfort symptoms.

3. Chamomile: The sedative properties of chamomile are well-known. Additionally, it can calm the digestive tract by lowering inflammation and calming the gastrointestinal system's muscles. It is general knowledge that chamomile tea relieves cramping, gas, and indigestion symptoms.

4. Turmeric: It contains curcumin, which is a strong anti-inflammatory and antioxidant substance. As such, it can enhance digestion, lessen intestinal inflammation, and maintain a balanced gut flora. Black pepper and turmeric are frequently combined to increase the potency and absorption of turmeric.

5. Slippery Elm: For centuries, slippery elm has been used to relieve the lining of the intestines and stomach. For ailments like acid reflux and inflammatory bowel disease (IBD), it creates a protective layer that might lessen irritation and inflammation in the digestive system.

Five Well-Known Herbal Supplements for Healthy Digestive System

Apart from individual herbs, a number of herbal supplements have become well-known due to their extensive advantages for gut health. The following five well-known herbal supplements are frequently taken to promote digestive health:

1. Digestive Bitters: A mixture of bitter herbs, digestive bitters encourage the formation of bile and digestive enzymes. Dandelion, burdock, and gentian roots are common constituents. Digestive bitters can facilitate better nutrition absorption, lessen bloating, and facilitate better digestion.

2. Aloe Vera: Aloe vera has calming and restorative qualities. Its juice or gel can serve the digestive system in three basic ways including, lowering inflammation in the gut, supporting the healing of the intestinal lining, and enhancing digestion.

Aloe vera is frequently applied to reduce the symptoms of inflammatory bowel syndrome (IBS), acid reflux, and other digestive issues.

3. Licorice Root: Traditional medicine has utilized licorice root to address a variety of digestive problems. It has ingredients that support ulcer healing, shield the stomach lining, and lessen inflammation. A very good example of licorice root that is often used to promote gut health is deglycyrrhizinated licorice (DGL).

4. Fennel: The carminative qualities of fennel seeds aid in the reduction of gas and bloating. Additionally, they have the ability to relax the gastrointestinal tract's muscles, which lessens cramping and indigestion sensations. The health of the digestive system is frequently supported by fennel tea or supplements.

5. Marshmallow Root: It's a mucilaginous herb that coats the lining of the digestive tract to provide protection. It can lessen discomfort, relieve inflammation, and support the repair of the stomach lining. Many people use marshmallow root to treat the symptoms of inflammatory bowel disease (IBD), gastritis, and acid reflux.

Five Vital Tips to Aid Safety and Efficacy of Herbal Supplements

Although there are many advantages to using herbal supplements for gut health, it's important to give attention to their safety and efficacy. Here are five important things to observe:

1. Seek Professional Counsel: It's important to see a healthcare practitioner before starting an herbal supplement regimen, particularly if you take medication or have any secondary diseases. It's possible for some herbs to interfere with drugs, or make particular medical disorders to become worse.

2. Quality and Purity: To guarantee purity and efficacy, select premium herbal supplements from reliable companies. Seek for goods that follow good manufacturing principles (GMP) and have undergone contamination testing.

3. Dosage and Usage: Adhere to the suggested dosage and usage guidelines on the label of the supplement or as instructed by your physician. Certain herbs can have negative consequences if used in excess.

4. Allergic Reactions: Recognize that certain herbs may cause allergic reactions. Stop using the product and get medical help if you encounter any symptoms of an allergic reaction, such as itching, rash, or respiratory distress.

5. Individual Reactions: Remember that every person may react differently to herbal supplements. An individual may not have the same results from something that works well for another person. You should take note of your body's reactions to herbal supplements and make necessary modifications.

Finally, herbal supplements provide a holistic and all-natural way to boost gut health. These herbs have a long track record of traditional use, and there is mounting scientific evidence to support their potential as useful assistants in enhancing digestive health. It is imperative to exercise caution when using them, consult healthcare professionals for advice, and select high-quality items. You can be proactive in establishing a healthy and balanced digestive system by including herbal medicines.

CHAPTER SEVEN

The Fundamentals of Bone Broth and Collagen as A Gut Health Product

Collagen and bone broth are two potent supporters in the pursuit of optimal gut health. This chapter will cover the positive effects of bone broth on gut health, the positive effect of collagen on gut health, and some of the top collagen and bone broth products on the market.

Five Positive Effects of Bone Broth on Gut Health

Animal bones and connective tissues are churned to create bone broth, which is a nutrient-dense liquid that has been ingested for generations. Its many health benefits — especially for gut health — have contributed significantly to its recent reawakening.

1. High in Nutrients: Vitamins, minerals, and amino acids are just a few of the vital nutrients that bone broth is full of. It also comprises easily absorbable minerals like calcium, phosphorus, magnesium, and other trace minerals.

2. Promotes Digestive Health: Gelatin, a disintegrated form of collagen, is an ingredient in bone broth. Gelatin has the ability to bond to water, making food pass through the digestive system more quickly. This can support the healing and protection of the digestive tract's mucosal lining, helping to treat ailments including leaky gut syndrome or increased gut permeability.

3. Anti-Inflammatory Properties: Glycine and arginine, two amino acids present in bone broth, have potent anti-inflammatory properties. Gastrointestinal health problems are frequently caused by chronic inflammation, which can be lessened and recovery can be encouraged by ingesting bone broth.

4. Joint Health: By preserving the wholeness of cartilage, the rubbery substance that cushions bones at joints, the collagen in bone broth promotes joint health. This effect is especially helpful for people with osteoarthritis and other related illnesses.

5. Immune Support: The immune system is favorably influenced by the positive effects of bone broth. There is a close relationship between the immune system and the gut, and a strong immunological response is influenced by a healthy gut. Bone broth is a great supplement to your diet since it contains minerals that boost immune system function in general.

Five Positive Effects of Collagen on Gut Health

Collagen is the highest abounding the human body. It is the protein that gives framework to bones, skin, nails, connective tissues, and hair. Collagen is also essential for preserving the health of the gut.

1. Strengthens the Lining of the Gut: Collagen maintains the stomach lining's structural uniformity. Collagen's amino acids, especially glutamine, support the integrity of the digestive tract's mucosal lining and stave off diseases like leaky gut syndrome or increased gut permeability.

2. Promotes a Healthy Inflammation Reaction: The anti-inflammatory qualities of collagen can aid in the healing and calming of the gut lining. Numerous digestive problems can result from persistent inflammation in the gut, however collagen might lessen these consequences.

3. Encourages Healthy Digestion: The gelatin that is obtained from collagen assists in the disintegration of proteins and calms the gut lining, which enhances digestion and the absorption of nutrients. General gut health and performance can be increased as a result of this effect.

4. Enhances Gut Flora: Collagen can support the upkeep of a balanced population of gut microbes. This effect is essential for general health since a well-balanced gut flora positively impacts immunity, digestion, as well as mental health.

You may get all of these advantages that have been listed in this chapter so far, and even more by including premium bone broth and collagen products in your diet. The following options are generally used:

Three Main Products for Bone Broth

1. Kettle & Fire Bone Broth: This rich, savory bone broth is produced from organic ingredients and the bones of cattle reared on grass. Kettle & Fire Bone Broth contains lots of collagen, gelatin, and amino acids, and it promotes immunological function, joint health, and gut health.

2. Bonafide Provisions Organic Bone Broth: Slow-simmered to extract optimum nutrients, this broth is prepared from organic, free-range chicken bones. Rich in collagen, protein, and minerals, Bonafide Provisions Organic Bone Broth eases inflammation and supports gut health.

3. Pacific Foods Organic Bone Broth: This easily portable and highly nutritious bone broth comes in chicken and beef variants. Rich in protein and minerals, it promotes gut health and general well-being.

Three Main Products for Collagen

1. Vital Proteins Collagen Peptides: It comes from the hides of pasture-raised, grass-fed bovine animals, and it's easily digestible, dissolving readily in both hot and cold beverages. This product promotes healthy joints, skin, hair, and nails as well as gut health.

2. Ancient Nutrition Multi Collagen Protein: It is fashioned out of a combination of collagen derived from four different food sources, including eggshell membranes, fish, chicken, and beef. This product offers extensive advantages for supporting joints, skin elasticity, and gut health.

3. Further Food Collagen Peptides: It is fashioned out of hydrolyzed collagen peptides, and it's prepared to be easily absorbable and bioavailable. This product helps to maintain healthy skin and joints, lower inflammation, and improve gut health.

In summary, collagen and bone broth are critical elements for preserving and perfecting gut health. They are a vital component of any gut health program due to their many advantages, which range from lowering inflammation to assisting the gut lining. You can make major progress toward optimal gut health by including collagen products and premium bone broth in your diet.

CHAPTER EIGHT

The Fundamentals of Anti-Inflammatory Foods as A Gut Health Product

The body's immune system naturally reacts to damage or illness by causing inflammation. Acute inflammation is necessary for healing, but persistent inflammation can cause a number of illnesses, such as cancer, autoimmune diseases, and digestive problems. The gut is especially susceptible to persistent inflammation since it is the home of billions of bacteria and an essential component of the immune system. Crohn's disease, ulcerative colitis, and Irritable Bowel Syndrome (IBS) can all be brought on by an inflamed gastrointestinal tract.

Inflammation management is largely dependent on healthy gut flora. Short-chain fatty acids (SCFAs), which have anti-inflammatory qualities and support the wholeness of the gut lining, are produced by beneficial bacteria in the gut. Conversely, dysbiosis, or an imbalance in gut flora, can lead to inflammation and jeopardize gut health. Inflammation levels and gut bacteria are significantly influenced by diet. By including foods that have anti-inflammatory properties in your diet, you can improve your gut health by managing and reducing chronic inflammation.

The Top Ten Anti-Inflammatory Foods for Gut Health

1. Fatty Fish: Omega-3 fatty acids are abundant in fatty fish, including sardines, mackerel, and salmon. Strong anti-inflammatory benefits are widely recognized for omega-3 fatty acids. It has been demonstrated to aid diseases like Crohn's disease

and inflammatory bowel syndrome (IBS) by assisting in the reduction of inflammatory molecule synthesis.

2. Berries: Antioxidants such as anthocyanins are abundant in berries, such as raspberries, strawberries, and blueberries. These substances counteract damaging free radicals, assisting in the reduction of inflammation. Additionally, berries encourage the development of useful gut bacteria known as probiotics.

3. Leafy Greens: Rich in vitamins, minerals, and antioxidants, leafy greens include spinach, kale, and Swiss chard. Essentially, leafy greens contain lots of vitamins A, C, and K that give them anti-inflammatory properties. In addition, fiber from these greens helps maintain a balanced microbiota in the gut.

4. Turmeric: Curcumin, a potent anti-inflammatory substance, is found in turmeric. Curcumin effectively reduces inflammation in the gut by inhibiting inflammatory pathways throughout the body. When black pepper is added to turmeric, it increases the absorption of curcumin.

5. Nuts and Seeds: They are famous sources of fiber, antioxidants, and healthy fats. Some examples of nuts and seeds are flaxseeds, chia seeds, walnuts, and almonds. They contain prebiotic fiber that feeds useful gut bacteria or probiotics, aiding in the reduction of inflammation and promotion of gut health.

6. Olive Oil: Oleic acid, which is a monounsaturated fat that has anti-inflammatory properties is found in extra virgin olive oil. Additionally, it has polyphenols, which are antioxidants that assist in lowering inflammation. Olive oil promotes a healthy gut flora and helps shield the lining of the gut.

7. Ginger: The bioactive molecule gingerol, which has anti-inflammatory and antioxidant qualities, is found in ginger. It can ease the symptoms of digestive issues including bloating and nausea by reducing inflammation in the gut.

8. Garlic: For generations, people have utilized garlic for its therapeutic benefits. Sulfur compounds found in it have anti-inflammatory properties. Additionally, garlic can assist in lowering inflammation in the gut, as well as encouraging the growth of probiotics, which are useful gut bacteria.

9. Green Tea: Packed with polyphenols, especially epigallocatechin gallate (EGCG) that possesses potent anti-inflammatory properties. Green tea consumption supports a healthy gut flora and assists in lowering inflammation.

10. Fermented Foods: Probiotics can be found in fermented foods such as miso, yogurt, kefir, sauerkraut, and kimchi. These advantageous bacteria lessen inflammation and provide a balanced gut flora. Additionally, fermented foods improve immune system health and nutrient absorption.

Seven Vital Tips for Including Anti-Inflammatory Foods in Your Diet

1. Start with Breakfast: You may include berries in your morning meals by inserting them into yogurt, oatmeal, or smoothies. Also, you can use extra virgin olive oil instead of standard cooking oil to prepare scrambled eggs or pan-fried vegetables. You can always find a way to include fermented foods in your diet with little imagination.

2. Snack Wisely: Throughout the day, choose to eat nuts and seeds as snacks. Nuts like walnuts or almonds can help reduce inflammation and keep you feeling full. Try some fruit with a small amount of chia seeds spread on it.

3. Use a Variety of Leafy Greens: Include a range of leafy greens in your diet. Put Swiss chard in your soups, kale in your salads, and spinach in your omelets. Smoothies are a great way to add leafy greens for an added nutritional boost.

4. Use Herbs and Spices: Use anti-inflammatory herbs and spices to season your food. Incorporate turmeric into your rice recipes, stews, and soups. Add ginger to smoothies, drinks, and stir-fries. Add some garlic to your marinades, dressings, and sauces.

5. Select Fatty Fish: Strive to consume fatty fish at a minimum of twice a week. This group of fish, including mackerel, sardines, or salmon can always be prepared in various ways to be enjoyed as a tasty and nourishing meal choice, either grilled, roasted, or broiled. To boost their anti-inflammatory purpose, you can serve them with olive oil and some green vegetables.

6. Consume Green Tea: Choose green tea in place of sweetened beverages. Savor it warm or cold, and for added taste and vitamin C, squeeze in some lemon. Regularly consuming green tea might enhance your general health and help lower inflammation.

7. Savor Fermented Foods: Make sure your diet includes a range of fermented foods. Eat kefir or yogurt for breakfast or as a snack. For your salads and sandwiches, put in some sauerkraut or kimchi. Add miso to soups and sauces to increase useful bacteria or probiotics in the gut.

You may alleviate chronic inflammation, promote gut health, and enhance your general health by including these anti-inflammatory items in your diet. These dietary modifications don't have to be difficult to make, as little, consistent alterations can have a big impact eventually.

CHAPTER NINE

The Fundamentals of Water as A Gut Health Product

Hydration is essential for preserving general health, and it has a major effect on gut health in particular. Water, which makes up almost 60% of the human body, is essential for several physiological processes, such as digestion and nutrition absorption. Water helps in the disintegration of food, enabling nutrients to be absorbed more effectively. Additionally, it facilitates the easy passage of food through the digestive system, thereby reducing constipation and encouraging regular bowel movements.

The Five Basic Values of Water to the Health of the Gut

1. Digestion: Saliva is produced with the help of water and contains enzymes that start the breakdown of meals. Additionally, it aids in the release of gastric juices, which are required for the disintegration of food in the stomach.

2. Nutrient Absorption: Staying adequately hydrated guarantees that the nutrients in your food are well absorbed into your blood. Dehydration can hinder the absorption of nutrients, resulting in dietary deficits and associated health problems.

3. Inhibiting Constipation: Water helps to make stools loose and easy to pass. Hard stools can result from chronic dehydration and cause discomfort as well as other gut-related problems.

4. Preserving Gut Flora: Adequate hydration promotes a balanced population of gut microorganisms. This equilibrium can be upset by dehydration, which can impair immunity and cause digestive disorders.

5. Detoxification: Water aids in the removal of waste materials and toxins out of the body through feces and urine. This process of detoxification is essential to preserving optimum gut health.

Six Practical Ways to Consume Enough Water for Gut Health

There's more to staying well-hydrated than merely drinking water. The following six recommendations can help you stay properly hydrated for intestinal health:

1. Drink Plenty of Water: Although it's generally advised to consume eight glasses or 64 ounces of water every day, each person's requirements may differ depending on their age, gender, climate, and degree of physical activity.

2. Consume Hydrating Foods: Include foods high in water in your diet, such as oranges, tomatoes, cucumbers, and watermelon. These foods supply vital vitamins and minerals in addition to water.

3. Minimize Dehydrating Drinks: Limit the consumption of alcohol and caffeinated beverages since these substances may have diuretic properties that cause water loss.

4. Check Your Hydration Level: Be mindful of symptoms of dehydration, including foul-smelling urine, dry mouth, exhaustion, and lightheadedness. Aim for pale yellow urine as a reliable sign of sufficient hydration.

5. Stay Hydrated While Exercising: Drink more water before, during, and after physical activity to replace the fluids lost through perspiration.

6. Drink Water to Begin and End Your Day: Drink water to boost your metabolism in the morning, and drink water to help with overnight digestion and detoxification at night.

Five Common Hydration Products

Apart from ordinary water, there are many items intended to improve hydration and promote gut health:

1. Electrolyte Drinks: These beverages have important electrolytes such as magnesium, potassium, and sodium, assisting in sustaining fluid balance and promoting muscle function. To cut back on extra calories, choose products with less sugar.

2. Herbal Teas: In addition to helping you get enough fluids each day, herbal teas like ginger, peppermint, and chamomile tea also have the ability to soothe your stomach. They can lessen bloating and help with digestion.

3. Coconut Water: Rich in electrolytes by nature, coconut water is a great choice for hydration. It is a low-calorie and delightful substitute for sugar-filled beverages.

4. Hydration Powders and Tablets: Water that contains dissolved hydration powders or tablets improves hydration. They frequently have a combination of vitamins and electrolytes to increase energy and hydration, particularly after strenuous exercise.

5. Seasoned Water: You can improve the taste of water by seasoning it with fruits, vegetables, and herbs. Berries and basil, cucumber and lime, and lemon and mint are popular pairings. Not only does seasoned water taste fantastic, but it also adds more nutrients.

Finally, adequate hydration is essential for gut health since it affects bowel consistency, nutrition absorption, digestion, and the harmony of gut flora. You may promote your general comfort and gut health by including hydration-enhancing items in your routine and adhering to best practices for hydration. Bear in mind that maintaining proper gut health starts with drinking enough water.

CHAPTER TEN

Adopting A Better Lifestyle for A Perfect Gut Health

There are other factors besides diet that affect gut health. Our lifestyle decisions have a big impact on keeping our gut flora and digestive system in good shape. This chapter examines key lifestyle modifications that can support gut health at its best, emphasizing stress reduction, exercise, and sleep.

The Consequence of Stress on Gut Health

Your gut health might suffer greatly from prolonged stress. Stress can have a direct impact on the digestive system because of the gut-brain axis, a bidirectional communication link between the gastrointestinal tract and the brain. Stress can modify the balance of the gut flora, increase gut permeability (commonly referred to as 'leaky gut'), and disrupt gut motility. Digestive disorders like irritable bowel syndrome (IBS), inflammatory bowel disease (IBD), and other gut-related illnesses can result from these alterations.

Four Common Stress-Reduction Techniques

1. Mindfulness and Meditation: These two practices have been shown to dramatically lower stress levels. Methods like mindfulness meditation, deep muscle relaxation, and deep breathing can assist in soothing the mind and lessening the physical impacts of stress.

2. Yoga and Tai Chi: These age-old forms of relaxation and stress reduction incorporate physical postures, breathing techniques, and meditation. Research has indicated that consistent practice of tai chi and yoga can help gut health by lowering inflammation and stress.

3. Cognitive Behavioral Therapy (CBT): This form of behavioral therapy can assist in reframing unfavorable ideas and creating more constructive coping strategies. It works especially well for people with gut illnesses linked to stress, such as inflammatory bowel syndrome (IBS).

4. Engaging in Outdoor Recreation: Walking in the outdoors, gardening, or just spending time outdoors can all help lower stress and enhance mental health, which in turn benefits gut health.

The Influence of Exercise on Gut Health

Frequent exercise helps to keep the gut healthy in addition to improving cardiovascular health. By improving intestinal motility, exercise lowers the menace of constipation. It also assists in retaining a healthy weight, which is essential for preventing gut problems linked to obesity.

Four Major Types of Exercise for Gut Health

1. Aerobic Exercise: Heart rate is raised and cardiovascular health is enhanced by exercises including cycling, swimming, walking, and jogging. It has been demonstrated that aerobic exercise increases the variety of gut bacteria, an indication of fine gut health.

2. Strength Training: Including resistance training like weightlifting in your habit of physical fitness can support the maintenance of muscle mass and general body strength, which in turn supports a high-functioning metabolism and gut health.

3. Exercises for Flexibility and Balance: Exercises like yoga and Pilates not only help with flexibility and balance but lower stress as well, having an incidental effect on gut health.

4. Non-vigorous Intensity: It's critical to continue exercising at a moderate intensity. This is because, overtraining or excessive physical activity can have the opposite impact, possibly increasing inflammation and gut permeability or leaky gut.

The Influence of Sleep on Gut Health

Restorative sleep is necessary for the body's upkeep, particularly the digestive system. Insufficient sleep can cause the circadian cycle to be obstructed, which can have a detrimental effect on the gut flora and raise the danger of gastrointestinal problems.

Five Vital Tips for Enhancing the Soundness of Sleep

1. Establish a Routine: You can enhance the soundness of your sleep when you go to bed and wake up at the same time every day, owing to the regulation of your circadian rhythm or body's internal clock.

2. Establish a Calm Environment: Endeavor that your bedroom is calm, cold, and dark to promote restful sleep. Whenever necessary, think about utilizing earplugs, sound conditioners, or blackout curtains.

3. Reduce Screen Time: The hormone melatonin, which controls sleep, can be disrupted by the blue light that is emitted by computers, phones, and tablets. Endeavor to stay away from screens for a minimum of one hour before going to bed.

4. Good Sleep Practices: Steer clear of coffee and large foods right before bed. Before going to bed, try engaging in relaxation practices like mild yoga, having a warm bath, reading a book, or meditating.

5. Manage Stress: To keep stress from getting in the way of your sleep, include stress-reduction strategies into your everyday routine.

In summary, adopting these lifestyle modifications will go a long way in perfecting your gut health. You may maintain your gut flora and promote general digestive health and comfort by controlling stress, getting consistent exercise, and getting sound sleep. Always bear in mind that maintaining your gut health requires caring for both your physical and mental well-being.

CHAPTER ELEVEN

The Concept of Personalizing A Gut Health Strategy

Gut health is a vital aspect of human health in general, impacting both digestion, immunity, and mental health. You must first ascertain the existing condition of your gut in order to customize a plan for gut health. This entails evaluating a number of elements, such as your food choices, lifestyle, medical history, and digestive problems.

Four Aspects of Assessing Gut Health

1. Digestive Symptoms: Be mindful of symptoms including heartburn, gas, diarrhea, bloating, and constipation. These may be signs of dysbiosis in your gut flora.

2. Nutritional Practices: Assess your general diet composition, including how much fiber, probiotics, and prebiotics you consume.

3. Lifestyle Factors: Ponder over your stress levels, sleep patterns, exercise routines, and any possible current use of antibiotics, because they can all have a profound effect on gut health.

4. Medical History: Observe any allergies, long-term illnesses, or gastrointestinal problems that may have an impact on your gut health.

Four Essential Methods for Evaluating Gut Health

1. Symptom Journals: You can find routines and reasons by keeping a daily journal of your symptoms, food, and lifestyle.

2. Food Sensitivity Tests: A thorough food sensitivity examination can assist in identifying whether a particular food is causing gut problems.

3. Stool Tests: A thorough stool examination can reveal information on the harmony of bacteria in your gut, the existence of infections, and the effectiveness of your digestive system.

4. Getting Medical Assistance: A gastroenterologist or other healthcare specialist can provide expert assessments and suggest relevant tests.

Four Essential Elements of a Personalized Strategy for Ideal Gut Health

1. Dietary Adjustments: Include foods high in probiotics, such as fermented vegetables, yogurt, and kefir, as well as foods high in prebiotic fiber, such as onions, bananas, and garlic. Increase your consumption of both soluble and insoluble fibers by eating whole grains, legumes, vegetables, and fruits. Drink enough water to aid with digestion and the absorption of nutrients. To determine sensitivity, temporarily cut out suspected trigger foods like dairy, gluten, and FODMAPs or fermentable oligosaccharides, disaccharides, monosaccharides, and polyols, which are short-chain carbohydrates that are poorly absorbed in the small intestine.

2. Lifestyle Adjustments: Reduce stress, which can have a detrimental effect on gut health, by engaging in mindfulness, meditation, or yoga. Try to get between seven

to nine hours of good sleep every night to help your gut and general health. Exercise on a consistent basis to support proper digestion and a balanced gut flora.

3. Supplementation: Take into account a premium probiotic supplement made to fit your individual requirements. Enzyme supplements might aid in the more efficient breakdown of meals if you have digestive problems. Make sure you're getting enough vitamins and minerals to meet your nutritional needs, especially if you have dietary limitations.

4. Expert Advice: An expert can assist in creating a well-balanced diet and suggest the right supplements. A specialist's routine examinations can help you watch over your gut health and handle any issues.

Three Ways of Tracking Your Progress Toward Optimum Gut Health

1. Symptom Journals: Keep track of your dietary adjustments, lifestyle modifications, and symptoms. Make a note of any updates or newly discovered problems.

2. Frequent Check-Ins: Arrange routine assessments with your medical professional to gauge advancement and make required modifications.

3. Objective Measures: To monitor changes in your gut health objectively, use stool tests or other diagnostic tools on a consistent basis.

Three Steps to Modifying Your Strategy for Ideal Digestive Health

1. Flexibility: Be ready to modify your plan in light of your development. If some foods still cause problems, you might want to try cutting them out permanently.

2. Reintroductions: To gauge tolerance and pinpoint certain triggers, reintroduce foods one at a time.

3. Ongoing Education: To hone and enhance your strategy, and stay up to date on fresh discoveries and advancements in the field of gut health.

Three Steps to Maintaining Gut Health Over the Long Term

1. Sustainable Habits: Put your attention on adopting long-term lifestyle adjustments that promote gut health.

2. Preventive Care: Proactive treatment and routine examinations can help avert future problems with gut health.

3. Holistic Approach: Keep in mind that general well-being and gut health are related. To promote your gut and overall health, prioritize self-care, have a balanced diet, and minimize stress.

You can attain and sustain optimal gut health and improve your entire quality of life by evaluating your gut health, developing a personalized strategy, and regularly observing and modifying your strategy.

CONCLUSION

We have explored the complex and interesting realm of gut health all through this book. We've looked at the basic functions of digestive enzymes and probiotics, revealing their advantages and showcasing the best products that can help keep the gut healthy. We've also looked at the important connection between gut health and inflammation, highlighting anti-inflammatory foods that can help and improve your gut health. Our aim has been to give you a thorough understanding of the products and procedures that can assist you in achieving and preserving optimal gut health.

It takes an all-round strategy that combines a balanced diet, frequent exercise, stress reduction, and the use of specific supplements to achieve enduring gut health. The following six fundamental tactics are important to remember as you proceed on your path to perfecting your gut health:

1. Balanced Diet: To support the health of your gut flora, include a range of foods high in fiber, such as vegetables, fruits, legumes, and whole grains. Consume foods high in probiotics on a consistent basis, such as fermented vegetables, kefir, and yogurt, to keep your gut flora in balance.

2. Digestive Enzymes: You should think about using digestive enzyme supplements in your regimen if you have digestive problems. These can lessen distress and bloating by assisting your body in disintegrating food more effectively.

3. Anti-Inflammatory Foods: Eat foods like almonds, leafy greens, berries, and fatty fish on a regular basis to help reduce inflammation. These meals can improve total digestive health by lowering intestinal inflammation.

4. Hydration: To ensure that your digestive system runs well, drink a lot of water. Preserving the intestinal mucosal lining and fostering the right balance of beneficial bacteria depend on adequate hydration.

5. Exercise: Work out frequently to strengthen the muscles in your digestive system and encourage regular bowel motions. Additionally, the health of the gut is promoted by stress reduction that results from exercise.

6. Stress Management: Long-term stress has a deleterious effect on gut health. Engage in stress-relieving practices like meditation, yoga, deep breathing techniques, or just spending time outdoors.

Undertaking the pursuit of perfecting your gut health is a worthy and useful venture. Be aware that every action you do to strengthen your gut health is an action that will improve your general health. Perseverance will be necessary for your success because noticeable changes might not happen right away. Pay attention to your body, modify as necessary, and consult a specialist when required.

The condition of your gut is highly relevant to your general health, impacting almost everything concerning the health of your body, ranging from your immune system to your mental health. You will be facilitating a better, happier future when you endeavor to make practical use of the products and procedures that were discussed in this book. Remain inquisitive, knowledgeable, and, above all, dedicated to your journey toward perfect gut health.

ABOUT THE AUTHOR

James Edwards was born on May 16th, 1974. He suffered from schizophrenia in the year 1998, which threatened to ruin his mental health. It happened that when James Edwards was miraculously healed of his mental sickness in the year 2012, he decided to serve mankind with his mental prowess. He does rigorous research on relevant subject matters and documents his discoveries in the form of concise and clear short nonfiction books.

"FINANCIAL LITERACY FOR TEENS AND YOUNG ADULTS" is one of his popular books. Other books include "UNDERSTANDING MEDICAL TERMINOLOGY BY MASTERING PREFIX AND SUFFIX," "LOWER CHOLESTEROL NATURALLY," and "A SHORT DESCRIPTION OF THE SECRET OF RELIEVING PAIN BY TRAINING YOUR NERVOUS SYSTEM DIFFERENTLY." He is a prolific author of plenty of short nonfiction books. Every word James writes is infused with his genuine desire to positively impact every reader's life and his passion for personal progress.

Start reading James Edwards's books now to begin your road toward a more purposeful and happy existence.

You can discover his other useful and highly interesting short books by visiting his author central page here: https://www.amazon.com/author/jamesedwards1974

www.ingramcontent.com/pod-product-compliance
Lightning Source LLC
Chambersburg PA
CBHW051709250726

48653CB00007B/2934